Paleo Slow Cooker Recipes

79 Delicious, Easy and Healthy Slow Cooker Recipes for the Paleo Diet

Copyright © 2013 by Pam Taylor
All rights reserved. This book or any portion thereof may not be reproduced or used in any manner whatsoever without the express written permission of the publisher except for the use of brief quotations in a book review.

Printed in the United States of America.
First Printing, 2013

Table of Contents

Introduction 2

Condiments 8

Homemade Mustard 9

Homemade Mayonnaise 10

Homemade Slow Cooker Ketchup 12

Homemade Slow Cooker Worcestershire Sauce 14

Homemade Slow Cooker Barbecue Sauce. 15

Homemade Slow Cooker Barbecue Sauce. 15

Appetizers 17

Apple Sausages with Mustard Sauce 18

Sausage Nutty Stuffed Mushrooms 19

Hot Wings 21

Spicy Cajun Pecans 23

Savory Barbecue Shrimp 24

Herb Mushrooms 25

Party Meatballs 27

Easy Barbecue Wings 29

Sides 30

Garlicky Mashed Cauliflower & Carrots 31

- Baked Sweet Potatoes 32
- Coconut Sweet Potato Casserole 33
- Seasoned Spaghetti Sauce 35
- Zucchini Noodles 36
- Bacon & Macadamia Sweet Potatoes 37
- Savory Butternut Squash 39
- Paleo Veggie Curry 40
- Delicious Spaghetti Sauce 42
- Pecan, Coconut & Apricot Acorn Squash ... 43
- Paleo Caponata 44
- Orange Herb Sweet Potatoes 46
- Savory Drumsticks 47
- Coconut Summer Squash 49
- Balsamic Herb Carrots 50
- Soups & Stews 51
- Garlic Chicken Soup 52
- Chicken Sweet Potato Stew 53
- Italian Kale Soup 55
- Creamy Tomato Soup 57
- Beef & Pumpkin Spice Stew 59
- Thai Coconut Milk Soup 61
- Rainy Day Stew 63

- Beef & Mushroom Soup 65
- Winter Beef Stew 67
- Pork Squash-Apple Stew 69
- Halibut & Sweet Potato Chowder 71
- Turkey Stew 73
- Yam & Basil Soup 74
- Slow Cooker Hot & Sour Soup 75
- Paleo Lamb Stew 77
- Beef & Cabbage Soup 78
- Chicken Vegetable Soup 79
- Tomato, Chicken & Herb Soup 81
- Dinners 83
- Barbecue Ribs 84
- Beef Bourguignon Paleo Style 85
- Meatballs in Marinara Sauce 87
- Roast Pork Dinner 89
- Zucchini Carbonara 91
- Lemon-Garlic Whole Chicken 93
- Egg & Veggie Casserole 95
- Artichoke-Mushroom Chicken 97
- Slow Cooker Pork Carnitas 99
- Stuffed Spaghetti Squash 101

- Creamy Cod & Carrots 103
- Cube Steak Supreme 105
- Shredded Pork & Apples 107
- Slow Cooker Cajun Turkey 109
- Sunday Night Roast Beef Dinner 110
- Herbed Salmon with Citrus 111
- Wild West Casserole 112
- Chicken & Vegetable Dinner 115
- Chicken Cacciatore Casserole 117
- Jambalaya Dinner 119
- Slow Cooker Ratatouille 121
- Steamed Tilapia Fillets 123
- Beanless Turkey Chili 124
- Sunday Roast Shredded Beef Wraps 125
- Savory Chicken Asian Style 126
- Creamy Tomato Zucchini Lasagna 128
- Desserts 130
- Walnut Cinnamon Apples 131
- Honey Chocolate Pears 132
- Fruit Compote with Toasted Macadamia Nuts 133
- Apple Apricot Crisp 135

Chocolate Coconut Tapioca Pudding 136
Paleo Bananas Foster with Toasted Coconut
.... 138

Introduction

Thank you for purchasing this cookbook! I am confident you will love these Paleo slow cooker recipes. Slow cooking is a great way to create wonderful dishes without a lot of effort. These Paleo recipes include:

Condiments

Sides

Soups & Stews

Main Dishes

And Even... Desserts

The Paleo Diet is commonly called the Cave Man Diet as it is centered around foods that our ancestors presumably lived on. The diet was first introduced in the mid 1970's by a gastroenterologist named Walter L. Voegtlin, who suggested the diet could help with digestive problems. Since that time it has become widely popular, with testimonials from numerous people claiming the diet has helped them in many areas, including:

Weight loss

Balanced blood sugar levels

Increased energy

Deeper sleep (more restful nights)

Clear skin

The Paleo way of eating takes thinking about food a little differently. Main stream advice about nutrition is opposite of what this diet recommends. Foods such as grains, which are a staple in many homes in the world, are not allowed on the Paleo diet. Learning to eat this way requires a different set of rules. If you're just starting the diet, the recipes in this book will help make the transition a little easier.

Foods the diet encourages you to avoid:

Processed foods

Refined foods

Dairy

Grains

Legumes

Foods the diet encourages you to eat:

Lean meats (grass-fed and cage-free are best)

Wild-caught fish and seafood

Eggs (from cage-free chickens)

Nuts and Seeds

Fruits

Most Vegetables
Healthy Fats

Explanation of some of the ingredients used in these recipes:

Even though it isn't listed in each recipe, I always recommend organic meats such as grass-fed beef, free-range and cage-free chicken and organic pork, which means the animals have had no hormones administered to them, and they are able to graze in organic pastures and eat organic grains. I also use wild-caught fish and seafood, as farm raised fish are full of chemicals and are very unhealthy.

The sweeteners I use are raw honey, which has anti-viral, anti-bacterial and anti-fungal properties; sucanut, which is a minimally refined sugar from cane juice that is darker in color because it retains some of the natural molasses; and evaporated cane juice, which is a less refined form of white sugar. It is made from sugar cane and retains a small amount of nutrients. Any kind of sugar, including fruit, is recommended to be eaten in moderation on the Paleo diet. I use extra virgin olive oil and extra virgin coconut oil in most of my cooking. However, there are other oils you can use on the Paleo diet that are equally as good for you. These include: flaxseed oil, sesame seed oil, avocado oil, macadamia nut oil, walnut oil, and other nut oils.

In place of dairy, I use almond and coconut milk which are both delicious and nutritious!

For seasoning, I use sea salt, freshly ground pepper, dried and fresh herbs, Bragg's Liquid Aminos (a certified non-GMO product that is derived from organic soybeans and can be used in place of soy sauce), and homemade Worcestershire sauce (recipe included).

Most vegetables are approved for the Paleo diet. Starchy vegetables such as potatoes, yams, corn and squash are allowed but hold less nutritional value, so eat these veggies in moderation. Most vegetables cook very well in the slow cooker. Some of the recipes include vegetables that are canned or frozen, but feel free to substitute fresh instead. Although eating Paleo takes finding new ways of cooking and enjoying food, the challenge can yield great results, including a healthier body!

Now that we've covered the basics, it's time for the recipes! Enjoy!

Condiments

When eating Paleo, it isn't necessary to give up your favorite condiments, especially if you make them yourself! Creating your own sauces is fun and definitely healthier as you can choose quality ingredients. The Mustard and Mayonnaise recipes are not slow cooker recipes. I decided to include them as they are used in some of the recipes in this book.

Homemade Mustard

3/4 cup mustard seeds (any variety)

2/3 cup white wine

2/3 cup white wine vinegar

1 medium onion or 2 shallots, diced

1/8 tsp. ground allspice

Sea salt and pepper

Directions:

Combine all ingredients except salt and pepper in a bowl and stir well. Cover and refrigerate overnight. Place mixture in a blender and puree to desired consistency. Season to taste with salt and pepper.

Homemade Mayonnaise

*There has been controversy over using raw eggs due to the risk of salmonella poisoning. For this reason, some people prefer to cook the egg yolks a bit in their mayonnaise recipes. Just so you have a choice, I'm including both the raw and cooked versions for this recipe.

4 large egg yolks

4 Tbsp. fresh lemon juice

4 Tbsp. homemade mustard

1/2 cup white wine vinegar

1 ½ - 2 cups olive oil

Sea salt

Directions:

Cooked Version:

In a small saucepan combine egg yolks, lemon juice, mustard and vinegar. Cook over low heat stirring constantly until mixture is slightly thickened. Remove from heat and pour into a blender. Allow to cool for 5 – 10 minutes. Start blender on Low. Slowly drizzle oil down the center hole into the egg mixture. Continue until mixture looks like mayonnaise. Season with salt and place in a container. Store in refrigerator for up to one week.

Raw Version:

Place egg yolks, lemon juice, mustard and vinegar in a blender; blend slightly to combine all ingredients. With blender on Low, slowly drizzle oil down the center hole until the mixture looks like mayonnaise. Season with salt and store in refrigerator.

Homemade Slow Cooker Ketchup

1 – 28 oz. can whole tomatoes

2 medium onions, chopped

2 stalks celery, chopped

4 garlic cloves, minced

2 Tbsp. grated fresh ginger

1 jalapeno or red chili pepper, ribs and seeds removed, minced

2 Tbsp. olive oil

2 tsp. ground coriander

1 tsp. dried fennel

1/2 cup chopped fresh basil

1 ½ cups vinegar (can be balsamic, apple cider, or red or white wine)

Sea salt and pepper

Directions:

Combine tomatoes, onion, celery, garlic, ginger, jalapeno or red chili pepper, olive oil, coriander, fennel and basil in a 4 – 5 qt. slow cooker. Cover and cook on High for 1 – 2 hours. Add vinegar and continue to cook, uncovered, until sauce reaches desired consistency. Using an immersion blender, puree sauce until smooth. Season to taste with salt and pepper. Let cool, put in a container and store in refrigerator.

Homemade Slow Cooker Worcestershire Sauce

1 cup raw apple cider vinegar

1/4 cup water

2 garlic cloves, smashed

4 Tbsp. Bragg's Liquid Aminos

1/2 tsp. ground ginger

1/2 tsp. ground mustard

1/2 tsp. onion powder

1/4 tsp. ground cinnamon

Sea salt and pepper

Directions:

Combine all ingredients in a 3 – 4 qt. slow cooker. Cover and cook on High for 1 – 2 hours or until mixture is boiling. Remove garlic and let cool. Pour into a container and store in the refrigerator.

Homemade Slow Cooker Barbecue Sauce

4 cups homemade ketchup

1 medium onion, diced

4 garlic cloves, minced

6 Tbsp. olive oil

1/2 cup white or red wine vinegar

2/3 cup homemade Worcestershire sauce;

2/3 cup raw honey

1 Tbsp. chili powder

1/2 tsp. ground cumin

1/4 tsp. ground thyme

1/4 tsp. cayenne pepper

Sea salt and pepper

Directions:

Combine all ingredients in a 4 – 5 qt. slow cooker. Cover and cook on Low for 4 – 5 hours. Uncover and continue cooking for 2 – 3 hours or until sauce is at desired consistency. Season with extra salt and pepper if desired.

Appetizers

What's a party without delicious appetizers? These dishes are easy to throw together a few hours before the party starts and are ready when guests arrive.

Apple Sausages with Mustard Sauce

2 lbs. chicken apple sausage links, cut in chunks

1 medium onion, chopped

4 Tbsp. homemade mustard

4 Tbsp. balsamic vinegar

6 Tbsp. raw honey

Directions:

Place sausage slices and onion in a 4 - 5 qt. slow cooker. Combine remaining ingredients and pour over sausage. Cover and cook on Low for 4 - 6 hrs. Serve using toothpicks.

Serves 8 – 10

Sausage Nutty Stuffed Mushrooms

20 large mushrooms

1/2 lb. sausage

1 small red onion, very finely diced

2 cloves garlic, minced

1/2 tsp. sea salt

1/4 tsp. black pepper

1/2 tsp. paprika

1/4 cup almond butter

1/4 cup fresh parsley, finely chopped

Directions:

Clean mushrooms. Remove and chop stems; set aside. In a skillet, brown sausage. Add mushroom stems, onion and garlic; cook until onion is soft. Add sea salt, pepper, paprika, almond butter and parsley; mix well. Stuff each mushroom with about 1 Tbsp. meat mixture. Place in a 5 - 6 qt.

slow cooker. Cover and cook on High for 1 - 2 hrs.

Serves 8 – 10

Hot Wings

5 – 6 pounds chicken wings

2 Tbsp. olive oil

Sea salt and pepper

1 cup hot sauce

2 Tbsp. homemade Worcestershire sauce

1 jalapeno, ribs and seeds removed, finely diced

1/2 tsp. garlic powder

1/4 tsp. onion powder

Chopped fresh parsley

Directions:

In a bowl combine wings, olive oil, salt and pepper. Toss to coat. Pour wings out on a baking tray. Place under broiler for 5 – 6 minutes on each side. Remove from oven and place in a 4 – 5 qt. slow cooker. Combine hot sauce, Worcestershire sauce, jalapeno, garlic powder and onion powder; stir well and pour over wings. Cover and cook on

High for 2 – 3 hours or until chicken is cooked through.

Serves 6 – 8

Spicy Cajun Pecans

1 lb. pecan halves

1/4 cup olive oil

1 Tbsp. chili powder

1 tsp. hot sauce

1 tsp. dried basil

1 tsp. dried oregano

1 tsp. dried thyme

1 tsp. sea salt

1/2 tsp. onion powder

1/4 tsp. garlic powder

Directions:

Combine all ingredients in a 3 - 4 qt. slow cooker. Cover and cook on High for 20 min. Turn to Low and continue cooking, uncovered. Allow to cook stirring occasionally for 2 hrs. Pour nuts onto a baking sheet and allow to cool.

Serves 8 – 10

Savory Barbecue Shrimp

2 pounds large fresh shrimp, unpeeled

Sea salt and pepper

2 garlic cloves, minced

1/2 cup homemade barbecue sauce

2 Tbsp. homemade Worcestershire sauce

1 Tbsp. homemade mayonnaise

1 tsp. hot sauce

Juice of 1 lemon

Directions:

Place shrimp in a 5 – 6 qt. slow cooker; sprinkle with salt and pepper. Combine garlic, barbecue sauce, Worcestershire sauce, mayonnaise, hot sauce and lemon juice; pour over shrimp. Cover and cook on High for 1 hour or until shrimp turn opaque.

Serves 4 – 6

Herb Mushrooms

2 pounds fresh mushrooms, cleaned and sliced

1/4 cup olive oil

1/4 cup white wine

3 Tbsp. fresh lemon juice

2 garlic cloves, minced

1 tsp. sea salt

1 tsp. dried thyme

1/2 tsp. dried oregano

1/2 tsp. dried parsley

1/4 tsp. dried basil

1/8 tsp. onion powder

1/8 tsp. black pepper

Directions:

Place mushrooms in a 4 – 5 qt. slow cooker. Combine remaining ingredients and pour over mushrooms. Cover and cook on Low for 3 – 4 hours or until mushrooms are tender.

Serves 4 – 6

Party Meatballs

1/2 pound ground beef

1/2 pound Italian sausage

1 small onion, diced

1 garlic clove, minced

1 large egg

1/2 tsp. Italian seasoning

1/2 tsp. sea salt

1/8 tsp. black pepper

1 Tbsp. olive oil

1 ½ cups sweet chili sauce

1 Tbsp. fresh lemon juice

2 Tbsp. raw honey

Fresh chopped Italian parsley

Directions:

Combine the ground beef, sausage, onion, garlic, egg, Italian seasoning, salt and pepper; mix until combined. Place meatballs in a large skillet with olive oil; brown on all sides. Transfer meatballs to a 5 – 6 qt. slow cooker. Combine chili sauce, lemon juice and honey; pour over meatballs. Cover and cook on Low for 5 – 6 hours or until meatballs are thoroughly cooked. Sprinkle with fresh parsley and serve using toothpicks.

Serves 4 – 6

Easy Barbecue Wings

3 – 4 pounds chicken wings

1/2 tsp. garlic powder

1/2 tsp. onion powder

Sea salt and pepper

1 ½ cups homemade barbecue sauce

Directions:

Place wings on a baking sheet. Sprinkle with garlic powder, onion powder, salt and pepper. Place under broiler for 6 minutes. Turn wings over and broil another 6 minutes. Transfer wings to a 5 – 6 qt. slow cooker. Pour barbecue sauce over wings. Cover and cook on High for 1 – 2 hours or until wings are cooked through.

Serves 4 – 6

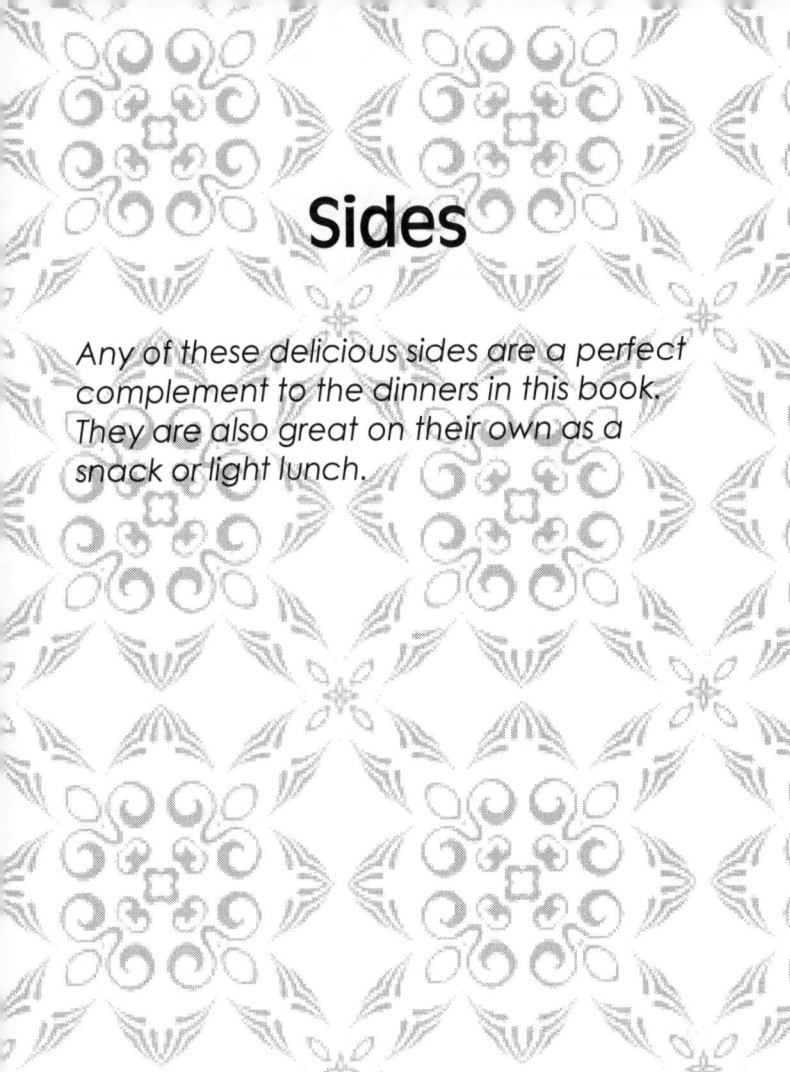

Sides

Any of these delicious sides are a perfect complement to the dinners in this book. They are also great on their own as a snack or light lunch.

Garlicky Mashed Cauliflower & Carrots

1 head cauliflower, chopped into pieces

2 carrots, chopped

2 garlic cloves

1/2 cup chicken broth

Sea salt and pepper

Directions:

Place cauliflower, carrots, garlic and chicken broth in and 3 – 4 quart slow cooker. Cover and cook on High for 1 – 2 hours or until vegetables are very tender. Spoon vegetables into a blender and blend until smooth. Season with salt and pepper.

Serves 4 – 6

Baked Sweet Potatoes

4 – 5 sweet potatoes

Coconut oil

Directions:

Rub coconut oil all over the sweet potatoes. Place in a 5 – 6 qt. slow cooker. Cover and cook on Low for about 6 hours or until sweet potatoes are soft.

Coconut Sweet Potato Casserole

4 cups mashed sweet potato (from Baked Sweet Potatoes)

1/4 cup coconut oil

1/4 cup raw honey

1/4 cup sucanut

2 large eggs

1 tsp. ground cinnamon

1/2 tsp. vanilla extract

1/2 tsp. maple extract

1/4 tsp. nutmeg

1/2 cup shredded coconut

1/2 cup coconut milk

Topping:

1 cup chopped pecans

1/2 cup sucanut

2 Tbsp. coconut oil

Directions:

Combine the sweet potato, coconut oil, honey, sucanut, eggs, cinnamon, vanilla extract, maple extract and nutmeg in a large mixing bowl. Mix until all ingredients are combined. Stir in shredded coconut and coconut milk. Pour mixture into a lightly greased 4 – 5 qt. slow cooker. Cover and cook on High 2 – 3 hours. Combine topping ingredients. Sprinkle over hot casserole.

Serves 6

Seasoned Spaghetti Sauce

1 medium spaghetti squash

1/2 cup water

Olive oil

Italian seasoning

Sea salt and pepper

Directions:

Cut spaghetti squash in half and scrape the seeds out. Set both halves, squash side down, in a 5 – 6 qt. slow cooker. Poke the tops of the squash with a fork several times. Pour in water, cover and cook on Low for 5 – 6 hours. Take squash out of the slow cooker (careful, it will be hot!) and scrape the squash away from the peel and put into a large bowl. Season with olive oil, Italian seasoning, salt and pepper.

Serves 4 – 6

Zucchini Noodles

2 – 3 medium zucchini squashes

1/2 tsp. dried parsley

Olive oil

Sea salt and pepper

Directions:

Using a julienne peeler, cut zucchini into long strips or noodles. Put in a 3 – 4 qt. slow cooker. Sprinkle dried parsley, olive oil and salt and pepper on top. Cover and cook on High for 2 – 3 hours or until noodles are tender.

Serves 4 – 6

Bacon & Macadamia Sweet Potatoes

1/2 pound bacon

1/2 cup chopped macadamia nuts

6 medium sweet potatoes, cut in chunks

1/4 cup vegetable broth

2 Tbsp. extra virgin coconut oil

1 Tbsp. ground cinnamon

1 tsp. ground cloves

1/2 tsp. allspice

1 tsp. sea salt

Directions:

In a skillet, fry bacon until crispy. Set on paper towel to drain and then put bacon and macadamia nuts in a container and set in fridge until the sweet potatoes are done. Place remaining ingredients in a 5 – 6 qt. slow cooker. Cover and cook on Low for 5 – 6 hours or until sweet potatoes are tender. Heat oven to 350. Pour batches of potatoes and liquids into a blender and blend until smooth. Put potatoes in a glass baking dish and sprinkle with the bacon and macadamia nuts. Bake at 350° for 20 – 30 minutes.

Serves 6 – 8

Savory Butternut Squash

2 medium butternut squashes, peeled and cubed

1 medium onion, diced

1 cup fresh sliced mushrooms

4 cups chicken broth

2 Tbsp. olive oil

2 Tbsp. lemon juice

1 tsp. Italian seasoning

Directions:

Place butternut squash, onion and mushrooms in a 4 – 5 qt. slow cooker. Combine chicken broth, olive oil, lemon juice and Italian seasoning; pour over vegetables. Cover and cook on Low for 6 – 8 hours.

Serves 6 – 8

Paleo Veggie Curry

2 medium sweet potatoes, peeled and cubed

4 carrots, sliced in rounds

1 cup fresh green beans, snipped in half

2 medium zucchini, chopped

1 medium onion, diced

3 garlic cloves, minced

1 – 14 oz. can diced Italian style tomatoes

2 cups chicken broth

2 tsp. curry powder

1 tsp. ground coriander

1/2 tsp. cinnamon

1/4 tsp. crushed red pepper flakes

Sea salt and pepper

Directions:

Combine all ingredients in a 5 – 6 qt. slow cooker. Cover and cook on Low for 6 – 8 hours or until vegetables are tender. Stir and serve.

Serves 6 – 8

Delicious Spaghetti Sauce

1/2 pound Italian sausage

1 medium onion, diced

1 small bell pepper, chopped

1 garlic clove, minced

2 – 24 oz. jars spaghetti sauce

1 cup fresh mushrooms, sliced

1 tsp. Italian seasoning

1 Tbsp. raw honey

Sea salt and pepper

Directions:

In a skillet brown the sausage. Add onions and cook until translucent. Add garlic and cook 1 minute. Transfer mixture to a 4 – 5 qt. slow cooker. Stir in remaining ingredients. Cover and cook on Low for 5 – 6 hours. Serve over zucchini noodles or spaghetti squash.

Serves 6 – 8

Pecan, Coconut & Apricot Acorn Squash

1 large acorn squash, cut in fourths, seeds removed

4 Tbsp. raw honey

2 Tbsp. coconut oil

1/4 cup chopped pecans

1/4 cup shredded coconut

1/4 dried apricots, cut in small pieces

1/8 tsp. sea salt

Directions:

Place acorn squash in a 5 – 6 qt. slow cooker, squash side up. Combine remaining ingredients; mix well. Spoon mixture into the hollow of each piece of squash. Cover and cook on Low for 6 – 7 hours or until squash is tender.

Serves 4 – 6

Paleo Caponata

1 medium eggplant, cubed

2 cups tomatoes, chopped in small chunks

2 small zucchini, cubed

1 small summer squash, cubed

4 stalks celery, sliced

1 medium onion, chopped

1/4 cup raisins

1 – 4 oz. can tomato paste

2 Tbsp. red wine vinegar

1 Tbsp. raw honey

1 tsp. dried parsley

Sea salt and pepper

1/4 cup chopped Kalamata olives

1/4 cup capers

Directions:

Combine all ingredients except for olives and capers in a 4 – 5 qt. slow cooker. Cover and cook on Low for 5 – 6 hours or until vegetables are tender. Add olives and capers and stir.

Serves 4 – 6

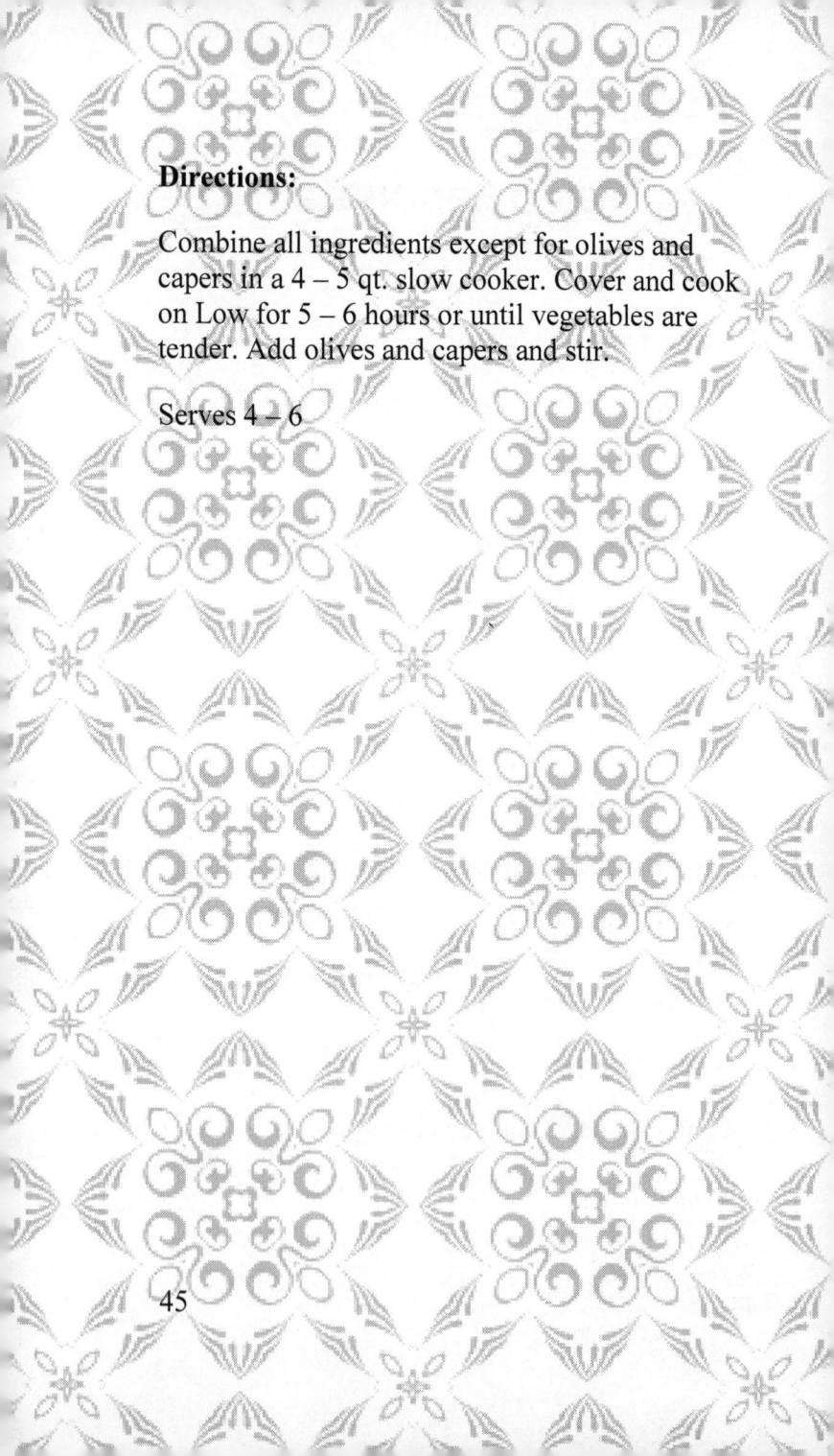

Orange Herb Sweet Potatoes

1/2 pound pancetta

5 medium sweet potatoes, peeled and cut in slices

1 cup orange juice

3 Tbsp. raw honey

1/2 tsp. Italian seasoning

1/2 tsp. dried sage

1/2 pound pancetta

Directions:

In a skillet sauté pancetta until crispy; put in a bowl and set in fridge. Place sweet potatoes in a 4 – 5 qt. slow cooker. Combine orange juice, honey, Italian seasoning and sage; pour over sweet potatoes. Cover and cook on Low for 5 – 6 hours or until sweet potatoes are soft. Garnish with pancetta.

Serves 6 – 8

Savory Drumsticks

6 pounds chicken drumsticks

1 small onion, diced

1 tomato, finely chopped

1 ½ cups sweet chili sauce

1/4 cup fresh lemon juice

1/4 cup blackstrap unsulphered molasses

2 Tbsp. homemade Worcestershire sauce

1 Tbsp. chili powder

1 tsp. garlic powder

Sea salt and pepper

Hot sauce

Directions:

Place drumsticks in a 5 – 6 qt. slow cooker. Combine onion, tomato, chili sauce, lemon juice, molasses, Worcestershire sauce, chili powder and garlic powder; stir well and pour over chicken. Sprinkle salt, pepper and hot sauce on top. Cover and cook on Low for 5 – 6 hours or until chicken is cooked through.

Serves 6 – 8

Coconut Summer Squash

3 medium summer squash, washed and sliced in rounds

1 medium onion, diced

1 – 14 oz. can coconut milk

Sea salt and pepper

Chopped fresh basil

Directions:

Place squash and onions in a 3 – 4 qt. slow cooker. Pour coconut milk over vegetables and season with salt and pepper. Cover and cook on High for 1 – 2 hours or until squash is tender. Garnish servings with fresh basil.

Serves 6 – 8

Balsamic Herb Carrots

3 pounds carrots, peeled and cut in strips

1 medium onion, cut in strips

1 Tbsp. raw honey

3 Tbsp. olive oil

2 Tbsp. balsamic vinegar

1/2 tsp. Italian seasoning

Sea salt and pepper

Fresh chopped Italian parsley

Directions:

Place carrots and onion in a 4 – 5 qt. slow cooker. Combine honey, olive oil, balsamic vinegar and Italian seasoning; pour over vegetables. Cover and cook on High for 3 – 4 hours or until carrots are tender. Season to taste with salt and pepper, and sprinkle with fresh parsley.

Serves 6 – 8

Soups & Stews

Who doesn't love a warm, comforting bowl of soup or stew? Try any of these delicious recipes on a cold day and your family will be thanking you!

Garlic Chicken Soup

3 chicken breasts, cut into pieces

1 large onion, chopped

4 carrots, sliced

4 stalks celery, sliced

1 cup fresh sliced mushrooms

8 cloves garlic, slightly mashed

1 tsp. Italian seasoning

1 – 6 oz. can tomato paste

1 cup chicken broth

Sea salt and pepper

Directions:

Place all ingredients except for salt and pepper in a 5 – 6 qt. slow cooker. Cover and cook on Low for 6 – 8 hours. Season to taste with salt and pepper.

Serves 4 – 6

Chicken Sweet Potato Stew

4 boneless skinless chicken breasts, cut in small chunks

1 small onion, chopped

2 stalks celery, chopped

3 sweet potatoes, peeled and cubed

3 carrots, peeled and sliced

1 – 28 oz. can stewed tomatoes

2 cups chicken broth

1 tsp. sea salt, or to taste

1 tsp. paprika

1 tsp. dried basil

1 tsp. celery seed

1/2 tsp. black pepper

1/8 tsp. cinnamon

1/8 tsp. nutmeg

Directions:

Combine all ingredients in a 4 - 5 qt. slow cooker; stir well. Cover and cook on Low for 6 - 8 hrs. or until chicken is cooked and vegetables are tender.

Serves 6 – 8

Italian Kale Soup

2 slices bacon, cut in 1/4 inch pieces

1/2 pound hot Italian sausage

1 medium onion, diced

2 garlic cloves, minced

4 cups chicken broth

3 small red potatoes, scrubbed and cut in slices

1 cup fresh sliced mushrooms

2 cups kale

1 cup coconut milk

Sea salt and pepper

Directions:

In a skillet fry the bacon until crispy; set aside. Using the same skillet, brown the sausage. Add onion and sauté until translucent. Add garlic and cook 1 minute. Transfer bacon and sausage mixture to a 5 – 6 qt. slow cooker. Add chicken broth, potatoes and mushrooms. Cover and cook on Low for 6 – 8 hours or until vegetables are tender. During the last hour of cooking time, add the kale, coconut milk, and salt and pepper to taste.

Serves 4 – 6

Creamy Tomato Soup

8 cups chopped fresh tomatoes

1 medium onion, diced

3 garlic cloves, minced

2 cups chicken broth

3 Tbsp. olive oil

2 tsp. Italian seasoning

2 Tbsp. tomato paste

1 Tbsp. raw honey

1 cup coconut milk

Sea salt and pepper

Chopped fresh Italian parsley

Directions:

Combine tomatoes, onion, garlic, broth, olive oil, Italian seasoning, tomato paste and honey in a 5 – 6 qt. slow cooker. Cover and cook on Low for 6 – 8 hours. Using an immersion blender, puree soup until smooth. Add coconut milk, salt and pepper to taste. Heat through. Garnish servings with fresh parsley.

Serves 6 – 8

Beef & Pumpkin Spice Stew

1 Tbsp. olive oil

1 large onion

1 pound cubed stew meat

4 cups cubed butternut squash

4 cups beef broth

2 tsp. ground sage

1 tsp. ground thyme

1 bay leaf

1 tsp. ground allspice

1/4 tsp. ground nutmeg

1 cup pumpkin, pureed

Sea salt and pepper

Directions:

In a skillet, heat the oil and sauté the onions until translucent. Remove onions and brown the stew meat on all sides. Place onions and meat in a 5 – 6 qt. slow cooker. Add the remaining ingredients except for pumpkin and salt and pepper. Cover and cook on Low for 6 – 7 hours or until the squash is tender. During the last 1/2 hour of cooking, add the pumpkin and salt and pepper to taste.

Serves 6 – 8

Thai Coconut Milk Soup

3 boneless, skinless chicken breasts, cubed

3 cups chicken broth

2 Tbsp. sweet chili sauce

1 Tbsp. chili garlic sauce

2 tsp. lemon grass paste

1 tsp. ginger paste

2 – 14 oz. cans coconut milk

2 – 4 oz. cans shiitaki mushrooms

1 – 15 oz. can baby corn

1 – 8 oz. can bamboo shoots

3 Tbsp. fish sauce

2 Tbsp. chopped fresh cilantro

1/4 cup sliced green onions

Lime wedges

Directions:

In a 5 – 6 qt. slow cooker combine cubed chicken, broth, sweet chili sauce, chili garlic sauce, lemon grass paste and ginger paste. Cover and cook on Low for 5 hours or until chicken is cooked. Add coconut milk, mushrooms, corn, bamboo shoots, fish sauce and cilantro. Cook 1 more hour. Garnish servings with green onions and lime juice.

Serves 8 – 10

Rainy Day Stew

1 lb. ground beef

1/2 lb. hot Italian sausage

1 onion, chopped

2 cloves garlic, minced

1 small head cabbage, shredded

3 ½ cups fresh diced tomatoes

2 cups tomato sauce

2 cups beef broth

2 tsp. raw honey

1/2 cup homemade Worcestershire sauce

1/2 tsp. Italian seasoning

Seasoned salt and pepper to taste

Directions:

In a skillet, combine ground beef and sausage; cook until browned. Add onions and garlic; cook 3 - 5 min. Transfer to a 4 - 5 qt. slow cooker. Add remaining ingredients and stir well. Cover and cook on Low for 6 - 7 hrs.

Serves 6 – 8

Beef & Mushroom Soup

1 tsp. seasoned salt

1/2 tsp. ground black pepper

2 lbs. beef chuck, cut into large cubes

2 Tbsp. olive oil

2 cups button mushrooms cut in half

4 red potatoes, scrubbed and cubed

2 carrots, peeled and sliced

2 beef bouillon cubes

1 cup dry red wine

3 cups beef stock

1 tsp. dried thyme

1/2 tsp. dried oregano

1/2 tsp. dried rosemary

1/2 tsp. onion powder

1 cup frozen peas

Sea salt and pepper to taste

Directions:

Combine flour, seasoned salt and black pepper. Dredge beef pieces in flour mixture. Heat oil in skillet and brown beef. Transfer to a 5 - 6 qt. slow cooker. Add mushrooms, potatoes and carrots. Dissolve bouillon cubes in red wine and beef stock; add spices. Pour over all. Cover and cook on Low for 8 - 10 hrs. Add peas during the last hour of cooking time.

Serves 8 – 10

Winter Beef Stew

2 – 3 pound chuck or flank steak, trimmed of any fat

3 garlic cloves, minced

Sea salt and pepper

1 medium onion, chopped

2 celery stalks, sliced

1 large bell pepper, chopped

1 cup winter squash, cubed

2 cups beef broth

1/2 cup red wine

2 tsp. ground cumin

1/2 tsp. dried oregano

Fresh chopped Italian parsley

Directions:

Place steak in a 5 – 6 slow cooker. Rub garlic over meat and sprinkle generously with salt and pepper. Place onions, celery, bell pepper and squash around meat. Combine beef broth, red wine, cumin and oregano; pour over meat and vegetables. Cover and cook on Low for 8 – 9 hours. Using two forks, slightly shred the steak. Serve garnished with fresh parsley.

Serves 4 – 6

Pork Squash-Apple Stew

2 Tbsp. butter

2 lb. pork tenderloin, cut in chunks

1 onion, chopped

2 cloves garlic, minced

3 cups cubed butternut squash

2 large cooking apples, peeled and cubed

3 potatoes, peeled and cubed

3 carrots, peeled and sliced

3 cups chicken stock

1 cup apple cider

2 tsp. sea salt

1/2 tsp. dried sage

1/2 tsp. dried rosemary

1/4 tsp. black pepper

1 bay leaf

Directions:

In a skillet, melt butter and brown pork on all sides. Transfer to a 5 - 6 qt. slow cooker. Add remaining ingredients and stir well. Cover and cook on Low for 6 - 8 hrs. or until vegetables are tender.

Serves 6 – 8

Halibut & Sweet Potato Chowder

5 slices bacon

1 medium onion, chopped

2 garlic cloves, minced

5 cups chicken broth

2 medium sweet potatoes, peeled and cubed

3 stalks celery, chopped

1 tsp. Italian seasoning

1/2 pound halibut, cut in chunks

1 – 14 oz. can coconut milk

Sea salt and pepper

Directions:

In a skillet, cook bacon until crispy. Add onion and garlic and sauté for 2 minutes. Transfer mixture to a 5 – 6 qt. slow cooker. Add broth, sweet potatoes, celery and Italian seasoning.

Cover and cook on High for 3 – 4 hours or until sweet potatoes are tender. Add halibut and coconut milk; cook for another hour. Season with salt and pepper.

Serves 6 – 8

Turkey Stew

2 cups cooked turkey breast, cubed

2 cups chicken stock

1 sweet potato, peeled and chopped

2 red potatoes, scrubbed and chopped

3 carrots, peeled and sliced

1 medium onion, chopped

1 cup frozen peas

1 cup sliced mushrooms

1 tsp. dried thyme

1 tsp. celery seed

Sea salt and pepper

Directions:

Combine all ingredients in a 4 - 5 qt. slow cooker; stir well. Cover and cook on Low for 4 - 6 hrs. or until vegetables are tender. Season to taste with salt and pepper.

Serves 6 – 8

Yam & Basil Soup

4 medium yams, peeled and cubed

1 medium onion, diced

2 garlic cloves, minced

1 – 14 oz. can coconut milk

2 cups chicken broth

2 tsp. dried basil

Sea salt and pepper

Fresh chopped basil

Directions:

Place all ingredients except for fresh basil in a 5 – 6 qt. slow cooker. Cover and cook on Low for 4 – 6 hours or until yams are soft. Using an immersion blender, blend soup until it reaches desired consistency. Garnish individual servings with fresh basil.

Serves 4 – 6

Slow Cooker Hot & Sour Soup

1/2 lb. pork tenderloin, sliced in thin strips

2 cups chicken stock

1 cup sliced mushrooms

1 – 8 oz. can sliced water chestnuts, drained

1 cup cubed firm tofu

1/2 cup bamboo shoots, sliced

2 Tbsp. Bragg's Liquid Aminos

2 Tbsp. rice wine vinegar

1 tsp. toasted sesame oil

1/4 tsp. crushed red pepper flakes

1 cup green onions, sliced

Directions:

Combine all ingredients except for green onion in a 4 - 5 qt. slow cooker. Cover and cook on Low for 6 - 8 hrs. or until pork is tender. Serve topped with sliced green onions.

Serves 6 – 8

Paleo Lamb Stew

2 pounds boneless leg of lamb, fat trimmed and cut in cubes

3 red potatoes, cut in chunks

4 carrots, sliced

1 sweet potato, peeled and cut in chunks

3 leeks, white part only, thinly sliced

3 stalks celery, thinly sliced

4 cups chicken broth

2 tsp. dried thyme

Sea salt and pepper

Chopped fresh Italian parsley

Directions:

Combine all ingredients except for fresh parsley in a 5 – 6 qt. slow cooker. Cover and cook on Low for 8 – 10 hours or until lamb is very tender. Garnish individual servings with fresh parsley.

Serves 6 – 8

Beef & Cabbage Soup

1 lb. lean ground beef

1 onion, chopped

2 garlic cloves, minced

2 carrots, peeled and sliced

2 stalks celery, chopped

1/2 head cabbage, shredded

1 – 6 oz. can tomato paste

1 Tbsp. homemade Worcestershire sauce

1 tsp. dried thyme

3 cups beef stock

Seasoned salt and pepper to taste

Directions:

In a skillet, brown beef with onion until thoroughly cooked. Place in a 4 - 5 qt. slow cooker. Add remaining ingredients and stir well. Cover and cook on Low for 6 - 8 hrs.

Serves 4 – 6

Chicken Vegetable Soup

3 lbs. chicken tenders

8 cups chicken broth

1 medium onion, chopped

2 stalks celery, chopped

2 carrots, sliced

2 cups cubed butternut squash

2 tsp. seasoned salt, or to taste

1 tsp. Italian seasoning

1 tsp. dried parsley

1/4 tsp. ground marjoram

1/4 tsp. black pepper

1 bay leaf

Directions:

Place chicken in a 5 - 6 qt. slow cooker. Add the rest of the ingredients. Cover and cook on Low for

6 - 8 hrs. Using two forks, shred chicken slightly. Stir and serve.

Serves 6 – 8

Tomato, Chicken & Herb Soup

1 Tbsp. olive oil

4 boneless skinless chicken thighs, cut in chunks

1 medium onion, chopped

3 garlic cloves, minced

6 cups chicken broth

2 cups diced tomatoes

1 small green chili, diced

1 10-oz. pkg. frozen chopped spinach, thawed and squeezed dry

2 Tbsp. chili powder

1 tsp. cumin

1/4 tsp. cayenne pepper

1 bay leaf

Salt and pepper to taste

Sliced green onions

Directions:

Heat oil in a skillet. Add chicken and cook until lightly browned. Transfer to a 5 - 6 qt. slow cooker. Add remaining ingredients, except for green onions. Cover and cook on Low for 6 - 8 hrs. Shred chicken using two forks. Serve topped with green onions.

Serves 6 - 8

Dinners

The best thing about most of these dinners is you can throw them together in the morning and by dinner time you have a hot, satisfying meal without a lot of fuss. Also, you can easily substitute just about any vegetable for the ones in these recipes. The slow cooker is very forgiving so feel free to experiment with your own combinations!

Barbecue Ribs

3 – 4 pounds pork ribs

Sea salt and pepper

1/2 cup white wine

1 Tbsp. homemade Worcestershire sauce

1 ½ cups homemade barbecue sauce plus more for serving

Directions:

Place ribs in a 5 – 6 qt. slow cooker; season with salt and pepper. Pour white wine around the meat. Combine the Worcestershire sauce and barbecue sauce; pour over ribs. Cover and cook on Low for 8 – 10 hours or until ribs are falling off the bone. Serve with additional barbecue sauce.

Serves 6 – 8

Beef Bourguignon Paleo Style

6 strips bacon, cut in 1-inch pieces

1 tsp. sea salt

1 tsp. pepper

4 lbs. beef chuck, cut in 2-inch cubes

1 onion, chopped

1 carrot, peeled and sliced

1 cup sliced mushrooms

2 cloves garlic, minced

1 Tbsp. tomato paste

2 cups red wine

1 cup beef broth

1/2 tsp. thyme

2 bay leaves

Directions:

In a skillet, sauté bacon until crisp; remove from skillet. Salt and pepper the beef and place in skillet with the bacon drippings. Brown beef on all sides. Transfer bacon and beef to a 5 - 6 qt. slow cooker. Add onion, carrot and mushrooms. Combine garlic, tomato paste, red wine, broth, thyme and bay leaves; pour over and around beef and veggies. Cover and cook on Low for 8 - 10 hrs. or until beef is very tender. You can serve this by itself as a stew or over hot Mashed Cauliflower and Carrots.

Serves 6 – 8

Meatballs in Marinara Sauce

1 pound ground beef

1 pound Italian sausage

1 small onion, diced

1 large egg

1/4 cup almond flour

2 garlic cloves, minced

2 tsp. Italian seasoning

1/2 tsp. sea salt

1/8 tsp. pepper

4 ½ cups fresh tomatoes, pureed

Directions:

In a large bowl, place the ground beef, sausage, onion, egg, almond flour, garlic, Italian seasoning, salt and pepper; mix until just combined. Shape into meatballs and place in slow cooker. Gently pour the pureed tomatoes over the meatballs.

Cover and cook on Low for 6 – 8 hours or until meatballs are tender.

Serves 6 – 8

Roast Pork Dinner

1 – 4 or 5 lb. pork roast

2 onions, chopped

4 carrots, sliced

1 cup chopped cauliflower

2 parsnips, sliced

1 cup red wine vinegar

4 garlic cloves, minced

1 Tbsp. crushed coriander seeds

1 Tbsp. crushed fennel seeds

1/2 tsp. sea salt

1/4 tsp. pepper

1 fresh rosemary sprig

3 dried bay leaves

Directions:

Place roast and onions in a 5 - 6 qt. slow cooker. Place carrots, cauliflower and parsnips around the roast. Combine remaining ingredients and pour over roast and veggies. Cover and cook on Low for 6 - 8 hrs. or until meat is tender.

Serves 8 – 10

Zucchini Carbonara

1/2 pound pancetta, diced small

1 small onion, diced

1 tsp. olive oil

2 medium zucchini squash

4 large eggs

1/4 cup whole coconut milk

3 garlic cloves, minced

Sea salt and pepper

Fresh chopped Italian parsley

Directions:

In a skillet, sauté the pancetta and onion in olive oil until onion is translucent; place in a 5 – 6 qt. slow cooker. Using a julienne peeler, take the zucchini and make long strips (noodles). Put noodles on top of the pancetta/onion mixture. Mix together the eggs, coconut milk, garlic and salt and pepper. Pour over noodles. Cover and cook on

Low for 4 – 5 hours, or until the zucchini noodles are tender. Garnish with fresh parsley.

Serves 4 – 6

Lemon-Garlic Whole Chicken

1 onion, chopped

1 – 5 to 6 lb. roasting chicken

1 lemon, cut in wedges

4 garlic cloves, slightly smashed

1 Tbsp. olive oil

1 Tbsp. sea salt

2 tsp. paprika

1 tsp. onion powder

1 tsp. cayenne pepper

1 tsp. dried thyme

1 tsp. white pepper

1/2 tsp. garlic powder

Directions:

Place the onion in the bottom of a 5 - 6 qt. slow cooker. Wash chicken and remove any giblets, etc. Stuff lemon and garlic into cavity. Place chicken on top of onions. Rub olive oil over chicken. Combine seasonings and rub them all over chicken. Cover and cook on Low for 6 – 8 hrs. Chicken will start falling off the bone when done. Serve as a roasted chicken dinner, or you can take the meat off the bones, freeze and use for several meals.

Serves 8 – 10

Egg & Veggie Casserole

Olive oil

8 large eggs

1/2 cup almond milk

1 pound sausage, broken up

1 medium sweet potato, grated

1 small red potato, grated

1 small onion, diced

1 cup fresh sliced mushrooms

1 small bell pepper, chopped

2 tsp. garlic powder

1 tsp. Italian seasoning

Sea salt and pepper

Directions:

Lightly grease a 5 – 6 slow cooker with olive oil. Beat the eggs with the almond milk and pour into cooker. Add the remaining ingredients in order shown. Cover and cook on Low for 7 – 8 hours. Cut in slices and serve.

Serves 8

Artichoke-Mushroom Chicken

2 cups whole artichoke hearts (canned)

2 cups sliced mushrooms

3 lbs. chicken tenders

1 cup marinated artichoke hearts

3/4 cup white wine

1/4 cup balsamic vinegar

2 Tbsp. olive oil

1/2 tsp. Italian seasoning

Sea salt and pepper to taste

Cooked spaghetti squash

Directions:

Place whole artichokes in a 5 - 6 qt. slow cooker. Top with mushrooms, then chicken. Pour marinated artichoke hearts (with liquid) over chicken. Combine wine, balsamic vinegar, olive oil, Italian seasoning, salt and pepper; pour over all. Cover and cook on Low for 4 – 6 hrs. Serve chicken mixture and sauce over hot cooked spaghetti squash.

Serves 8 – 10

Slow Cooker Pork Carnitas

3 pound pork shoulder

1 medium onion, diced

1 – 4 oz. can diced green chilies, mild

2 cloves garlic, minced

1 – 14 oz. can diced tomatoes

2 cloves garlic, minced

1/2 cup barbecue sauce

1 Tbsp. orange juice concentrate

Juice of 2 limes

1 Tbsp. raw honey

1 Tbsp. ground cumin

2 tsp. chili powder

2 tsp. onion powder

1/2 tsp. sea salt

1 medium avocado, mashed

1/2 cup salsa

Romaine lettuce leaves

Directions:

Place pork shoulder in a 5 – 6 qt. slow cooker. Add onion, green chilies and garlic. Combine barbecue sauce, orange juice concentrate, lime juice, honey, cumin, chili powder, onion powder and sea salt; pour over pork. Cover and cook on Low for 6 – 8 hours. Shred meat using two forks. Mix avocado and salsa together. Put some of the pork on a lettuce leaf and top with avocado salsa mixture.

Serves 6 – 8

Stuffed Spaghetti Squash

1 large spaghetti squash, halved lengthwise

1 – 14 oz. can Italian style diced tomatoes

3 – 6 oz. cans tuna in water, drained

1/3 cup sliced black olives

1 stalk celery, diced

2 Tbsp. homemade mayonnaise

2 tsp. homemade mustard

1 tsp. dried basil

1 tsp. Italian seasoning

Sea salt and pepper

Directions:

Place spaghetti squash (squash side up) in a 5 – 6 qt. slow cooker. Combine tuna, olives, celery, mayonnaise, mustard, basil and Italian seasoning; spoon into spaghetti squash. Sprinkle with salt and pepper. Cover and cook on Low for 6 – 8 hours, or until spaghetti squash is tender. Gently scrape squash and filling out onto a serving platter.

Serves 4 – 6

Creamy Cod & Carrots

3 pounds cod fillets

3 carrots, peeled and sliced in small rounds

1 small onion, diced

6 Tbsp. coconut oil

3 Tbsp. almond flour

1 Tbsp. homemade mustard

1/4 tsp. ground nutmeg

1 ½ cups coconut milk

Juice from 1 lemon

Sea salt and pepper

Directions:

Place cod, carrots and onion in a 5 – 6 qt. slow cooker. In a medium saucepan over medium heat, combine coconut oil, almond flour, mustard and nutmeg; whisk constantly while adding coconut milk until thickened slightly. Add lemon juice; pour over fish and vegetables. Sprinkle with salt and pepper. Cover and cook on High for 2 – 3 hours or until fish and vegetables are cooked.

Serves 4 – 6

Cube Steak Supreme

1 cup almond flour

1 Tbsp. sea salt

1 tsp. garlic powder

1 tsp. ground mustard

4 pounds cube steak

4 Tbsp. olive oil

1 medium onion, sliced

2 medium carrots, sliced

2 parsnips, sliced

1 beef bouillon cube

1 ½ cups water

Directions:

Mix together almond flour, salt, garlic powder and mustard. Dredge cube steak pieces in the flour mixture. Heat olive oil in a skillet. Place steaks in the oil and brown both sides. Add onion and sauté until soft. Transfer mixture to a 5 – 6 qt. slow cooker. Place carrots and parsnips around meat. Dissolve bouillon cube in water; pour around meat and vegetables. Cover and cook on Low for 6 – 8 hours.

Serves 6 – 8

Shredded Pork & Apples

2 pound pork shoulder

1 medium onion, diced

2 Fugi apples, peeled and cut in slices

1 cup chicken broth

2 garlic cloves, minced

2 Tbsp. fresh grated ginger

1 Tbsp. raw honey

1 tsp. ground cinnamon

1/2 tsp. paprika

1 bay leaf

Sea salt and pepper

Directions:

Put all ingredients in a 5 – 6 qt. slow cooker. Cover and cook on Low for 8 – 9 hours or until pork is falling apart. Shred pork using two forks.

Serve inside lettuce leaves or on top of hot cooked zucchini noodles.

Serves 4 – 6

Slow Cooker Cajun Turkey

4 turkey breasts

1 Tbsp. olive oil

1 Tbsp. onion powder

1 tsp. sea salt

1/2 tsp. ground black pepper

1/2 tsp. cayenne pepper

1/2 tsp. paprika

1/2 tsp. dried thyme

1/2 tsp. dried rosemary

1/4 tsp. ground nutmeg

1 cup chicken broth

Directions:

Place turkey breasts in a 4 - 5 qt. slow cooker; drizzle with olive oil. Combine seasonings and rub over turkey. Cover and cook on Low for 6 - 8 hrs. This makes an excellent roasted turkey to use for salads or soups.

Serves 6 – 8

Sunday Night Roast Beef Dinner

1 – 4 or 5 lb. chuck roast

1 Tbsp. beef bouillon

1/2 cup hot water

4 garlic cloves, minced

Sea salt and pepper

4 small red potatoes, quartered

4 carrots, peeled and sliced

2 cups cauliflower florets

1 red onion, cut in strips

Directions:

Trim fat from roast and place in a 5 - 6 qt. slow cooker. Dissolve bouillon in hot water; pour over roast. Spread minced garlic all over roast and sprinkle liberally with salt and pepper. Place vegetables around roast. Cover and cook on Low for 8 - 10 hrs. or until roast is very tender.

Serves 6 – 8

Herbed Salmon with Citrus

Large sheet of tin foil

3 – 4 pound salmon fillet

2 Tbsp. coconut oil

1/2 tsp. Italian seasoning

Sea salt and pepper

Juice of 1 lemon

Juice of 1 lime

1/4 cup fresh chopped Italian parsley

Directions:

Place salmon on the tin foil. Drizzle with coconut oil. Sprinkle with Italian seasoning, salt, pepper, lemon juice and lime juice. Fold foil around salmon and seal at edges; place in a 5 – 6 qt. slow cooker. Cover and cook on High for 2 hours. Garnish with Italian parsley and serve with steamed asparagus.

Serves 4 – 6

Wild West Casserole

1 1/2 lbs. ground beef

1 small onion, chopped

3 red potatoes, sliced in thin strips

2 sweet potatoes, peeled, cut in half and sliced in thin strips

1 – 14 oz. can diced tomatoes

2 Tbsp. almond flour

1/2 tsp. garlic powder

1/2 tsp. dried oregano

Sea salt & pepper to taste

Directions:

In a skillet, brown beef. Drain and place in a 4 - 5 qt. slow cooker. Sprinkle onions over beef, and then layer the potatoes and sweet potatoes on top. Combine tomatoes, almond flour, garlic powder, oregano, salt and pepper and pour over mixture. Cover and cook on Low for 6 - 8 hrs.

Serves 4 – 6

Chicken Lettuce Wraps

5 chicken breasts

Olive oil

Sea salt and pepper

4 Tbsp. Bragg's Liquid Aminos

2 Tbsp. apple cider vinegar

2 Tbsp. raw almond butter

1 Tbsp. raw honey

1 Tbsp. grated fresh ginger

1 Tbsp. Asian hot sauce of choice, or to taste

2 tsp. sesame oil

Sea salt and pepper

Washed lettuce leaves

Directions:

Place chicken in 5 – 6 qt. slow cooker. Drizzle with olive oil and sprinkle with salt and pepper.

Combine aminos, vinegar, almond butter, honey, ginger, hot sauce and sesame oil; mix well. Pour over chicken. Cover and cook on Low for 5 – 6 hours or until chicken can easily be shredded with two forks. Add salt and pepper to taste. Shred the chicken, place a small amount on a lettuce leaf and serve.

Serves 6 – 8

Chicken & Vegetable Dinner

4 boneless, skinless chicken breasts

Sea salt and pepper

1 – 15 oz. can crushed tomatoes

1 – 10 oz. pkg. frozen green beans

1 cup frozen corn

1 small onion, chopped

2 carrots, peeled and sliced

1 cup sliced mushrooms

1 garlic clove, minced

1/2 tsp. Italian seasoning

1 cup chicken broth

Directions:

Arrange chicken breasts in a 4 - 5 qt. slow cooker. Sprinkle with salt and pepper. Layer remaining ingredients over chicken. Cover and cook on High for 2 hrs. Reduce temperature to Low and continue cooking for 3 - 4 hrs.

Serves 4

Chicken Cacciatore Casserole

1/4 cup Italian dressing

3 lb. chicken thighs or drumsticks

1 large onion, chopped

1/2 cup chopped celery

1 cup fresh mushrooms, sliced

1/2 cup red pepper strips

1/2 cup green pepper strips

1 garlic clove, minced

1 14 1/2-oz. can crushed tomatoes

1 tsp. dried thyme

Spaghetti Squash, cooked

Directions:

In a skillet, heat dressing and add chicken. Brown on both sides. Place in bottom of a 4 - 5 qt. slow cooker. Layer onion, celery, mushrooms, red pepper, green pepper, garlic, tomatoes and thyme over chicken. Cover and cook on Low for 6 - 8 hrs. Serve over hot spaghetti squash.

Serves 8

Jambalaya Dinner

2 boneless skinless chicken breasts, cut into chunks

1/2 cup smoked sausage, sliced

1 bell pepper, chopped

1 onion, chopped

3 stalks celery, chopped

1 garlic clove, minced

1 14-oz. can diced tomatoes

2 Tbsp. chopped fresh parsley

1 tsp. dried thyme

1 tsp. dried oregano

1/2 tsp. sea salt

1/8 tsp. cayenne pepper

2 cups beef broth

1/2 lb. cooked, shelled shrimp

Directions:

Combine all ingredients except shrimp and rice in a 4 - 5 qt. slow cooker. Cover and cook on Low for 8 - 9 hrs. Increase temperature to High. Add shrimp and continue cooking 20 - 30 min. or until heated through.

Serves 4 – 6

Slow Cooker Ratatouille

2 large onions, sliced

3 medium zucchini, sliced

1 large eggplant, sliced

2 green bell peppers, cut is strips

6 large tomatoes, cut in small wedges

2 garlic cloves, minced

1 tsp. dried basil

2 tsp. sea salt

1/4 tsp. black pepper

2 Tbsp. chopped fresh parsley

1/4 cup extra virgin olive oil

1/4 cup toasted pine nuts

Directions:

Layer half of the onions, zucchini, eggplant, peppers, tomatoes and garlic in a 4 - 5 qt. slow cooker. Repeat once more. Sprinkle with basil, salt, pepper and parsley. Drizzle olive oil on top. Cover and cook on Low for 6 - 8 hrs. Remove lid and let sit for 10 min. before serving. Cut into serving pieces and top with toasted pine nuts.

Serves 6

Steamed Tilapia Fillets

Large sheet of tin foil

6 tilapia fillets

2 Tbsp. olive oil

1/4 tsp. dried thyme

1/4 tsp. garlic powder

Sea salt and pepper

Lemon wedges

Directions:

Place tilapia fillets on the tin foil. Drizzle with olive oil and sprinkle with thyme, garlic powder, salt and pepper. Wrap tightly in the foil and position so it can fit in a 5 – 6 qt. slow cooker. Cover and cook on High for 2 – 3 hours or until fish is flaky. Squeeze fresh lemon juice on servings and serve with steamed vegetables.

Serves 6

Beanless Turkey Chili

1 lb. ground turkey

1 onion, chopped

2 cloves garlic, minced

1 – 28 oz. can diced tomatoes

2 Tbsp. chili powder

2 tsp. cumin

2 tsp. salt

1/4 tsp. pepper

1 green bell pepper, chopped

Directions:

In a skillet, brown ground turkey until thoroughly cooked; add onions and garlic, cook for 2 - 3 min. Transfer mixture to a 4 - 5 qt. slow cooker. Add tomatoes and spices. Cover and cook on Low for 7 - 8 hrs. Add bell pepper during the last hour of cooking time.

Serves 4 – 6

Sunday Roast Shredded Beef Wraps

3 – 4 pound chuck roast, trimmed of fat

2 garlic cloves, minced

Sea salt and pepper

1 cup beef stock

1 sprig fresh rosemary

Romaine lettuce leaves

Homemade mayonnaise and mustard

Directions:

Place roast in a 4 – 5 qt. slow cooker. Rub garlic over entire roast and generously sprinkle with salt and pepper. Pour beef stock around the meat and set the rosemary sprig on top. Cover and cook on Low for 6 – 8 hours or until meat is falling apart. Using two forks, gently shred the roast. Spread some mayonnaise and mustard on a lettuce leaf. Put some of the meat in the leaf, roll tightly and serve.

Serves 4 – 6

Savory Chicken Asian Style

6 chicken breasts or 8 thighs, cut in chunks

3 cups fresh cubed pineapple

1 – 8 oz. can water chestnuts

1 medium onion, cut in strips

1 medium bell pepper, cut in strips

1/4 cup sliced green onions

2 cups chicken broth

3 Tbsp. Bragg's Liquid Aminos

2 Tbsp. fresh grated ginger

1 tsp. garlic powder

Sea salt and pepper

Directions:

In a 5 – 6 qt. slow cooker place chicken, pineapple, water chestnuts, onion, bell pepper and green onion. Combine broth, liquid aminos, ginger, garlic powder and salt and pepper; pour over vegetables. Cover and cook on Low for 6 – 8 hours or until chicken is cooked through.

Serves 6

Creamy Tomato Zucchini Lasagna

1 pound ground beef

1 medium onion, chopped

1 garlic clove, minced

1 cup sliced fresh mushrooms

1 – 28 oz. can crushed tomatoes

4 Tbsp. tomato paste

1/2 cup almond milk

1 tsp. Italian seasoning

2 medium zucchini, cut in long strips

Sea salt and pepper

Directions:

In a skillet brown ground beef; add onions, garlic and mushrooms and sauté until onions are translucent. In a bowl, combine crushed tomatoes, tomato paste, almond milk and Italian seasoning;

mix well. In a 5 – 6 qt. slow cooker, put a layer of the meat mixture, a layer of tomato mixture, a layer of zucchini and then season with salt and pepper; repeat until all ingredients are used. Cover and cook on Low for 6 – 8 hours, or until the vegetables are tender.

Serves 6 – 8

Desserts

Just because you're eating Paleo doesn't mean you can't enjoy dessert once in a while! These recipes will satisfy that nagging sweet tooth.

Walnut Cinnamon Apples

6 tart apples (Granny Smith works best), cored and tops cut slightly off

1/3 cup walnuts

1/3 cup sucanut

1 tsp. ground cinnamon

1/4 cup unsweetened apple juice

1 Tbsp. coconut oil

Directions:

Set apples in a 5 – 6 qt. slow cooker. Combine walnuts, sucanut and cinnamon. Spoon mixture into center of the apples. Pour the apple juice around the apples and drizzle coconut oil on top. Cover and cook on High for 2 – 3 hours or until apples are tender. Spoon some of the sauce from the slow cooker on top of the apples and serve.

Serves 6

Honey Chocolate Pears

8 firm pears (like winter or bosc pears), peeled and quartered

1/3 cup raw honey

3 Tbsp. cocoa powder

1 cup coconut milk

1/3 cup strong coffee

Directions:

Place pears in a 5 – 6 qt. slow cooker. Combine honey, cocoa powder, coconut milk and coffee; pour over pears. Cover and cook on Low for 2 – 3 hours or until pears are tender. Serve with sauce from the slow cooker drizzled over pears.

Serves 8

Fruit Compote with Toasted Macadamia Nuts

2 Gala or Fugi apples, peeled and cubed

2 medium firm pears, peeled and cubed

2 cups fresh pineapple chunks

2 cups pitted cherries

1/4 cup dried coconut

1/4 cup unsweetened apple juice

2 Tbsp. raw honey

2 Tbsp. sucanut

2 Tbsp. orange juice concentrate

2 Tbsp. quick-cooking tapioca

1 cup toasted macadamia nuts

Directions:

Combine all ingredients except for macadamia nuts in a 4 – 5 qt. slow cooker. Cover and cook on

High for 2 – 3 hours or until fruit is tender. Top individual servings with toasted macadamia nuts.

Serves 4 – 6

Apple Apricot Crisp

4 large Granny Smith apples, peeled and sliced

1 pound fresh apricots, pitted and cut in fourths

2 Tbsp. fresh lemon juice

1/2 tsp. ground cinnamon

Topping:

1/2 cup almond flour

1/2 cup shredded coconut

1/3 cup coconut oil

3 Tbsp. sucanut

1 cup chopped pecans

Directions:

Place apples and apricots in a 4 – 5 qt. slow cooker. Sprinkle with lemon juice and cinnamon; toss to coat. Combine almond flour, coconut, coconut oil and sucanut; mix well. Sprinkle over fruit. Cover and cook on High for 2 – 3 hours. Sprinkle pecans over individual servings.

Serves 6

Chocolate Coconut Tapioca Pudding

8 cups whole coconut milk

3/4 cup evaporated cane juice

3/4 cup pearl tapioca

3 large eggs

2 Tbsp. cocoa powder

1 tsp. vanilla extract

Directions:

Combine the coconut milk, evaporated cane juice and tapioca in a 4 – 5 qt. slow cooker; stir well. Cover and cook on High for 2 – 3 hours or until steaming. In a medium bowl whisk together eggs, cocoa and vanilla. Slowly pour some of the hot coconut milk mixture into the egg mixture while whisking constantly. Continue tempering the eggs until about 2 cups of the coconut mixture is used. Pour entire egg mixture back into slow cooker; stir well. Cover and cook an additional hour, then uncover and continue cooking until pudding is thickened to desired consistency. Delicious served warm or cold!

Serves 8 – 10

Paleo Bananas Foster with Toasted Coconut

6 bananas, peeled and sliced longways

5 Tbsp. coconut oil

3/4 cup sucanut

1/4 cup rum (optional)

1 tsp. vanilla extract

1 tsp. cinnamon

1/4 cup chopped pecans

1/4 cup toasted coconut

Directions:

Place bananas in a 5 – 6 qt. slow cooker. Combine coconut oil, sucanut, rum (if desired), vanilla and cinnamon; pour over bananas. Cover and cook on High for 1 hour. Sprinkle pecans and toasted coconut over bananas. Cover and cook for another 30 minutes.

Serves 6

Thank you for enjoying this cookbook!

Printed in Great Britain
by Amazon.co.uk, Ltd.,
Marston Gate.